A SEASON OF MEMORIES

AUTUMN

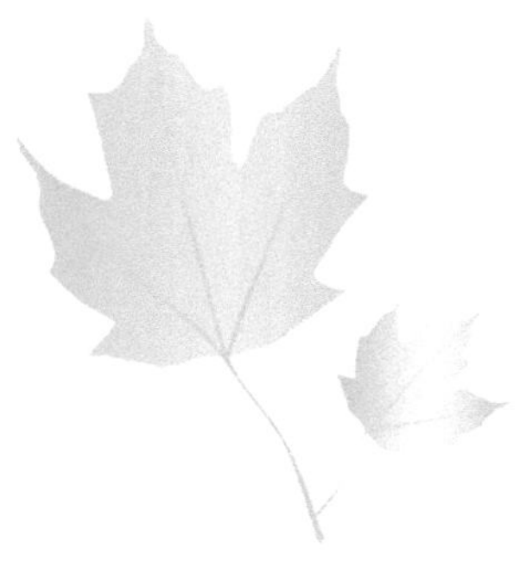

SUNNY STREET
BOOKS

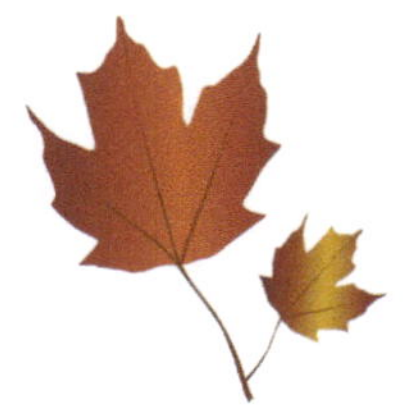

"When autumn came, my sister and I would rake fallen leaves into a big pile. Then we'd take a running jump and land right in the middle of them. It was so much fun!"

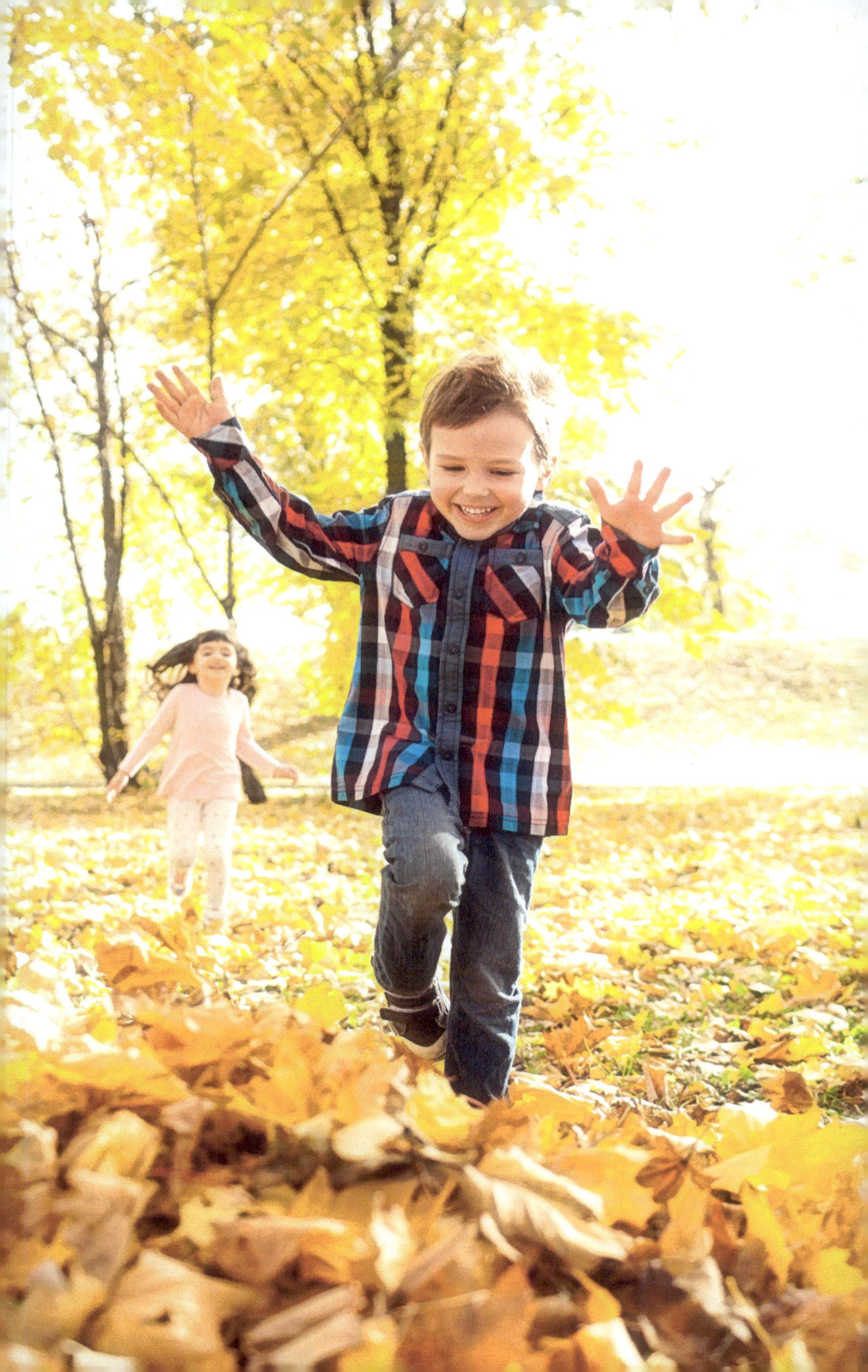

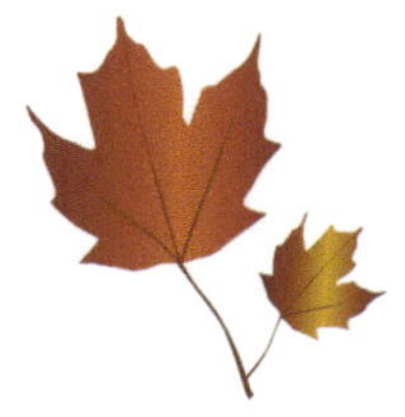

"When I was growing up, Halloween was always a big deal. One year my sisters and I went trick-or-treating dressed as witches. By the time we got home, our pumpkin baskets were filled with candy!"

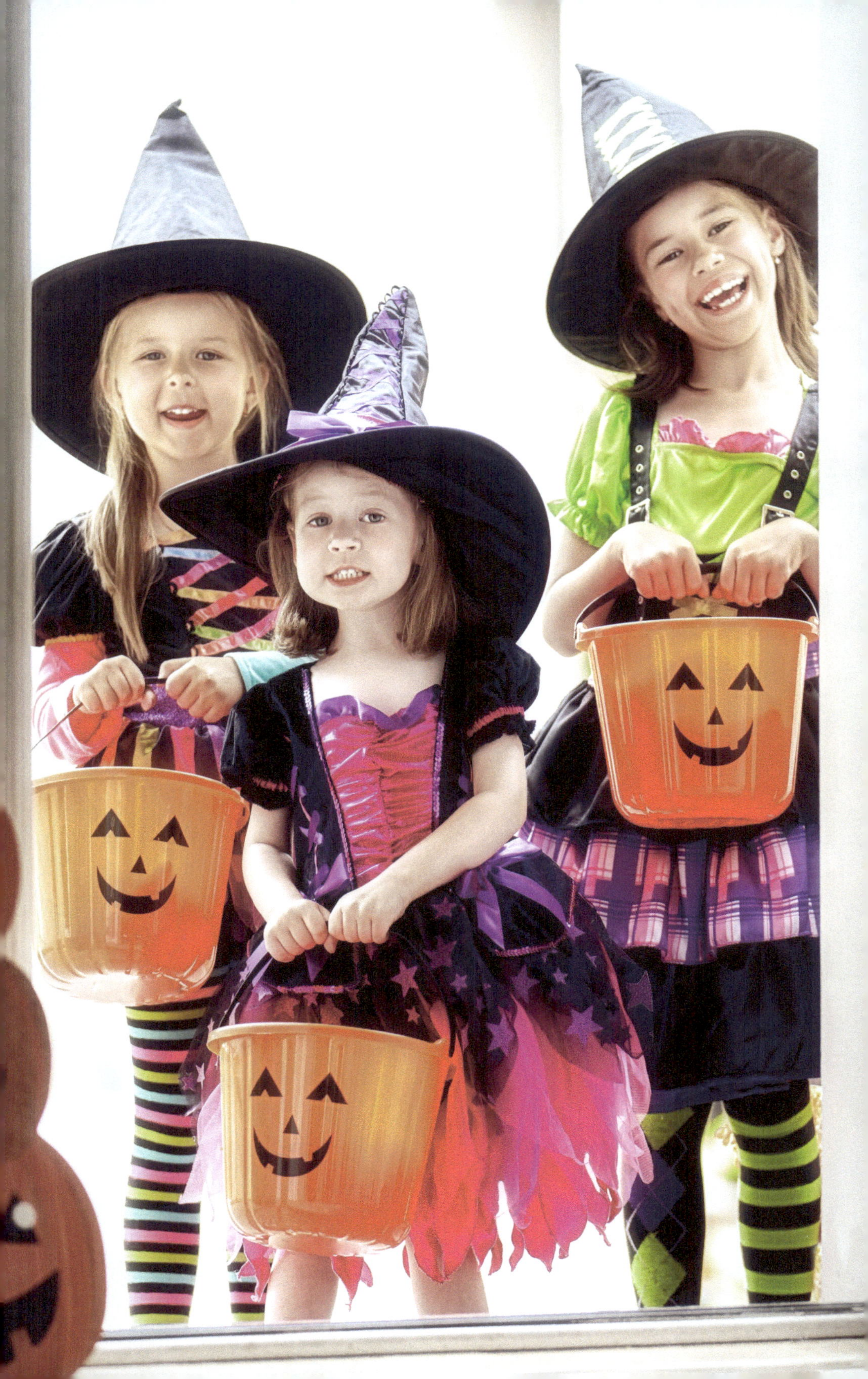

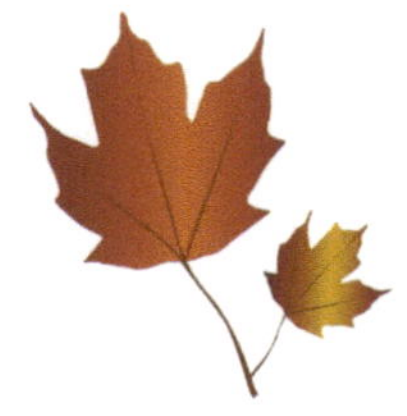

"When I was growing up, there was an apple orchard down the road from us. Every autumn we went there to pick apples. Then my Mom would make apple pie with ice cream on top!"

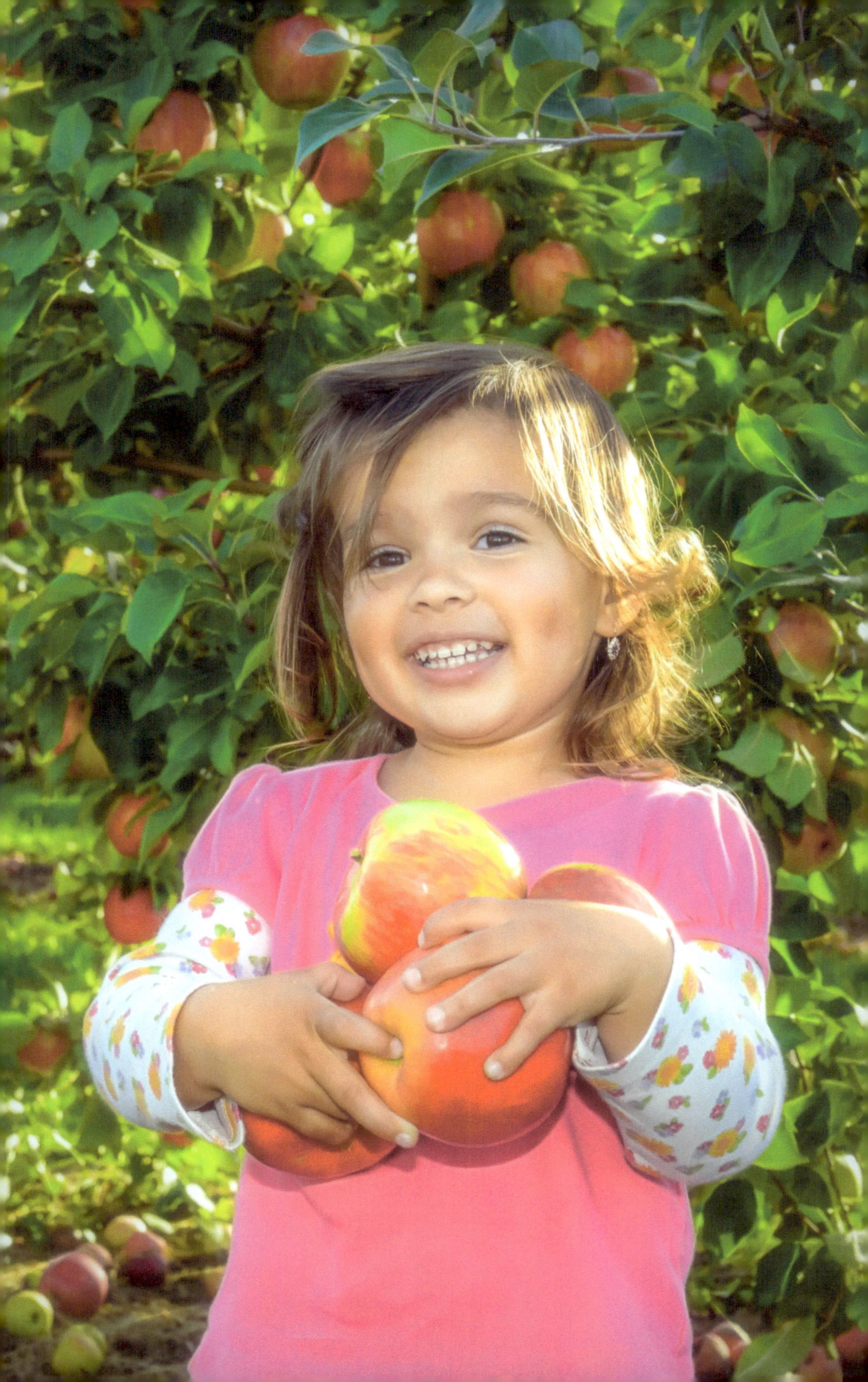

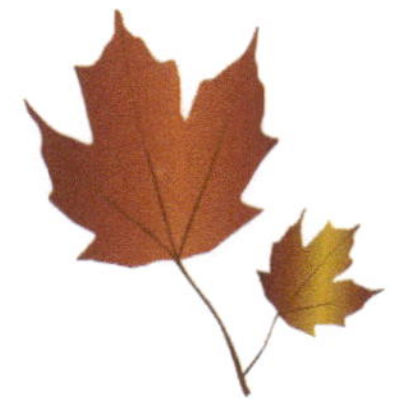

"My dog, Buddy, was my best friend. We loved taking long walks in the woods behind our house, especially when the summer heat gave way to cooler weather and the leaves turned beautiful autumn colors."

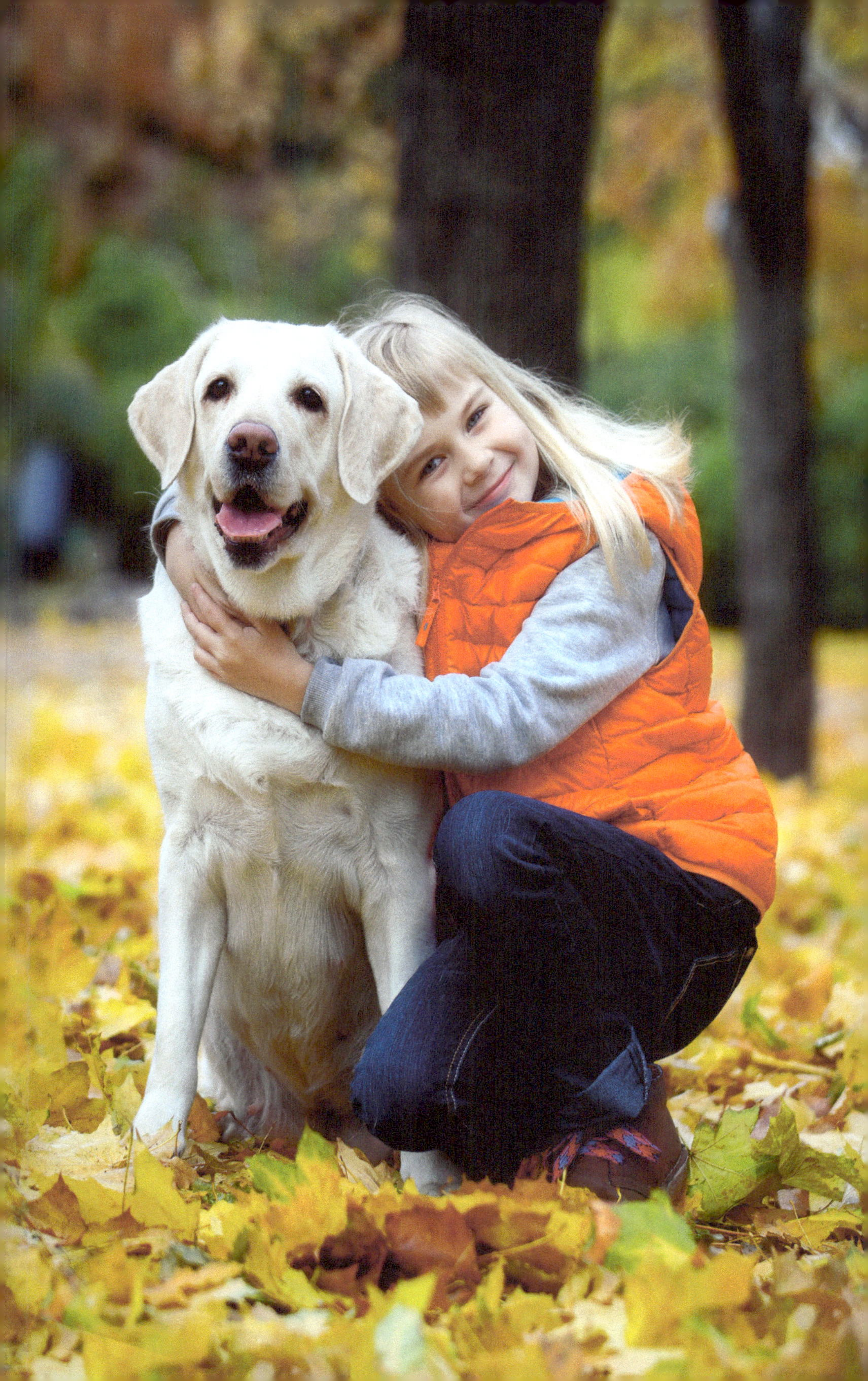

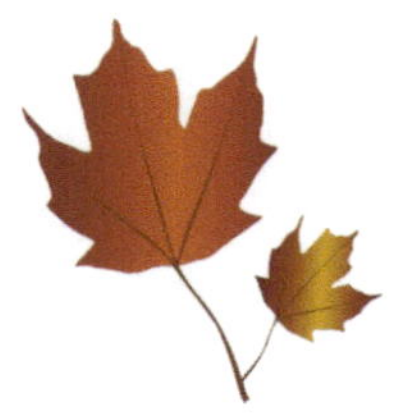

"It was a tradition in our
family every autumn to go to a
pumpkin patch. One year I found
the perfect pumpkin, but it was so
heavy I had to roll it all the way
to the front! Later we turned it
into the best Jack-O-Lantern we'd
ever had."

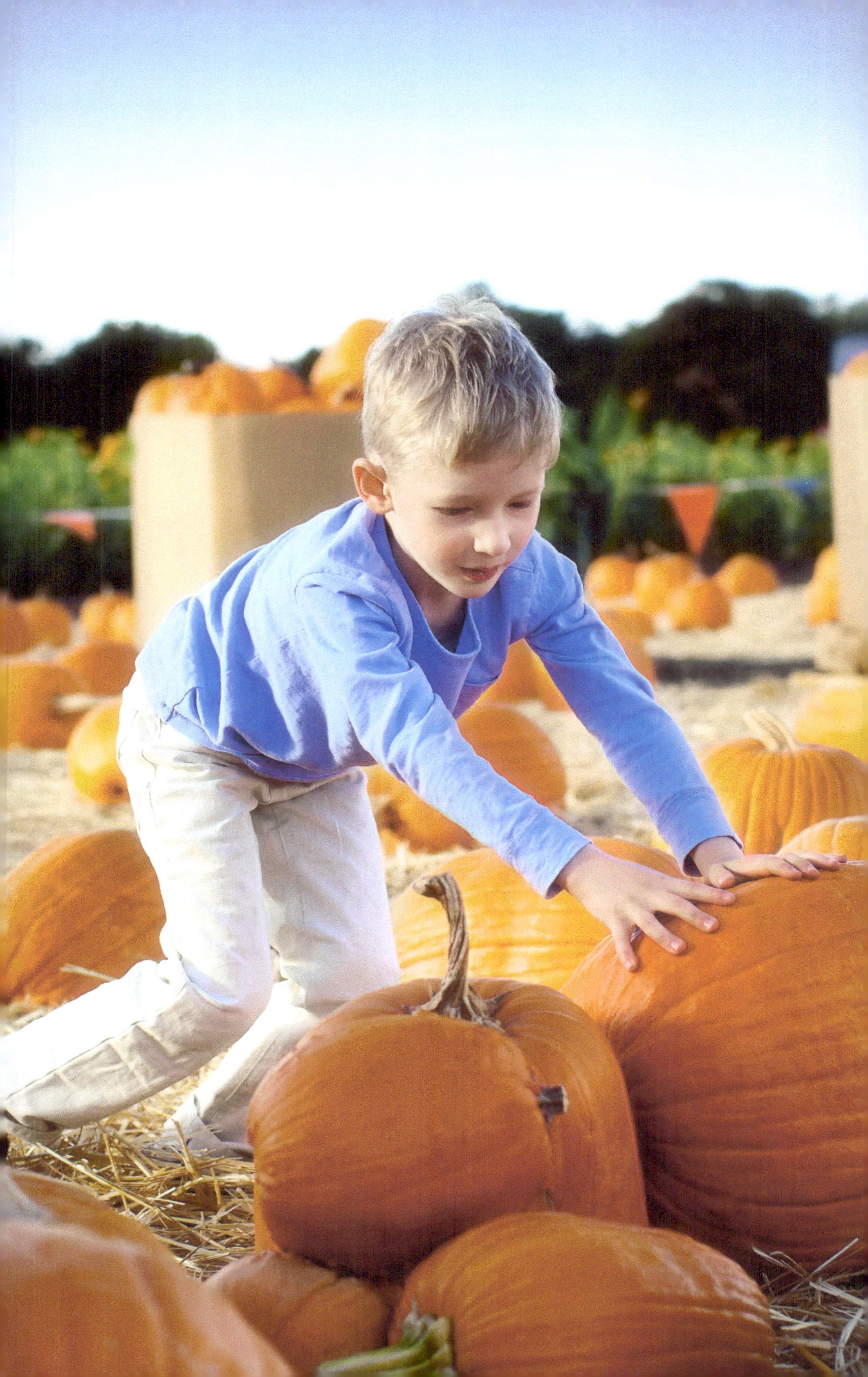

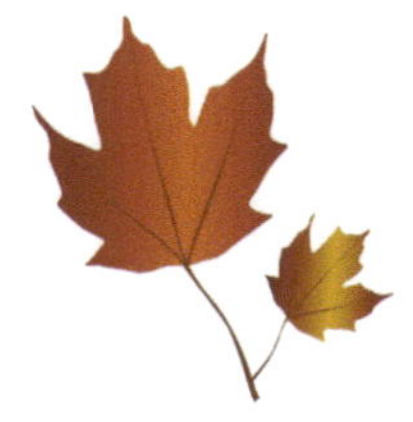

"I remember the year my Nana told me I was old enough to help with the Thanksgiving turkey. She showed me how to stuff it and prepare it for the oven. Later at dinner everyone said it was the best Thanksgiving turkey they'd ever had."

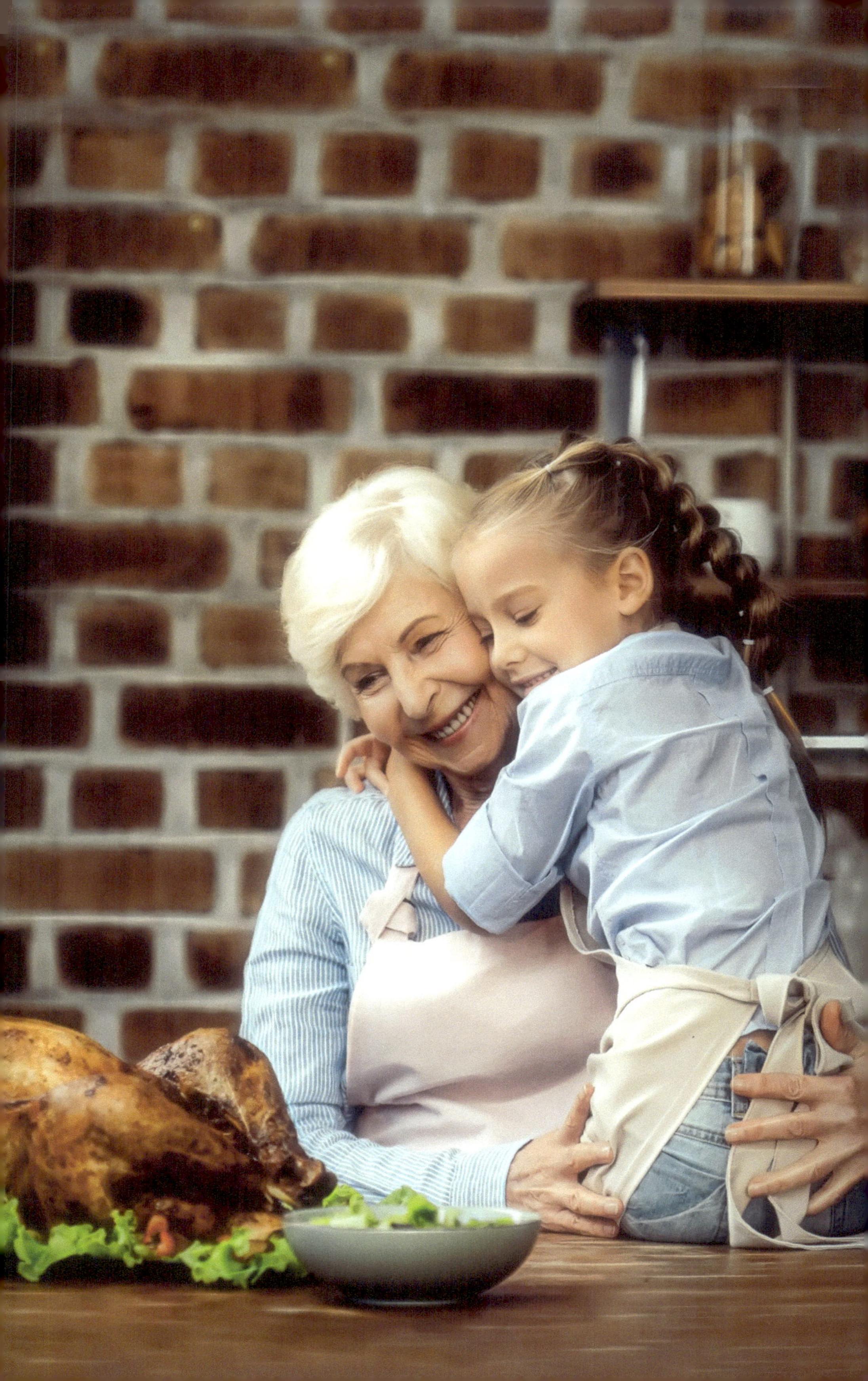

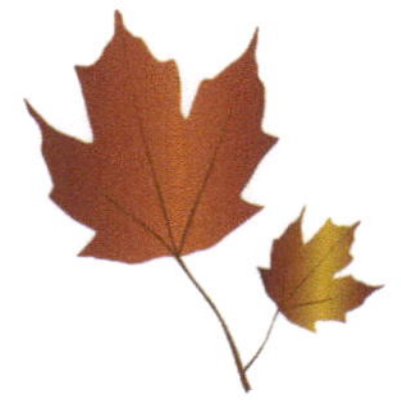

"When I was little, I found a gigantic leaf that had fallen from a tree in our front yard. I put it into a box and told my parents I never wanted to throw it away. Even though I'm all grown up now, I still have it. So maybe I really will keep it forever!"

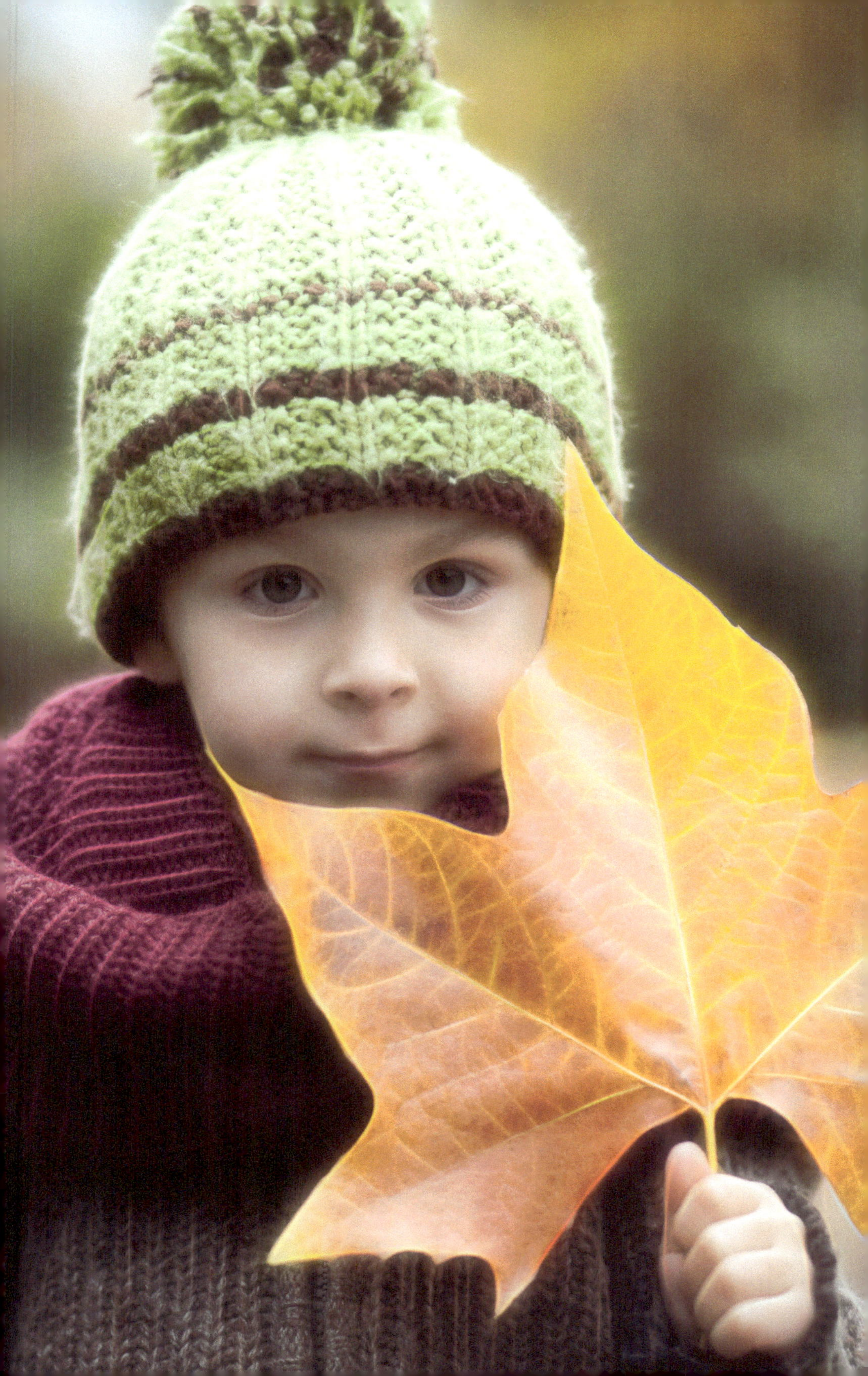

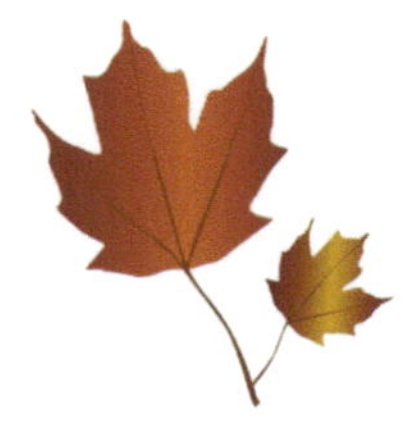

"My sister and I used to spend hours riding our bicycles through the nearby woods. I can still remember what our wheels sounded like as they crunched through the fallen leaves."

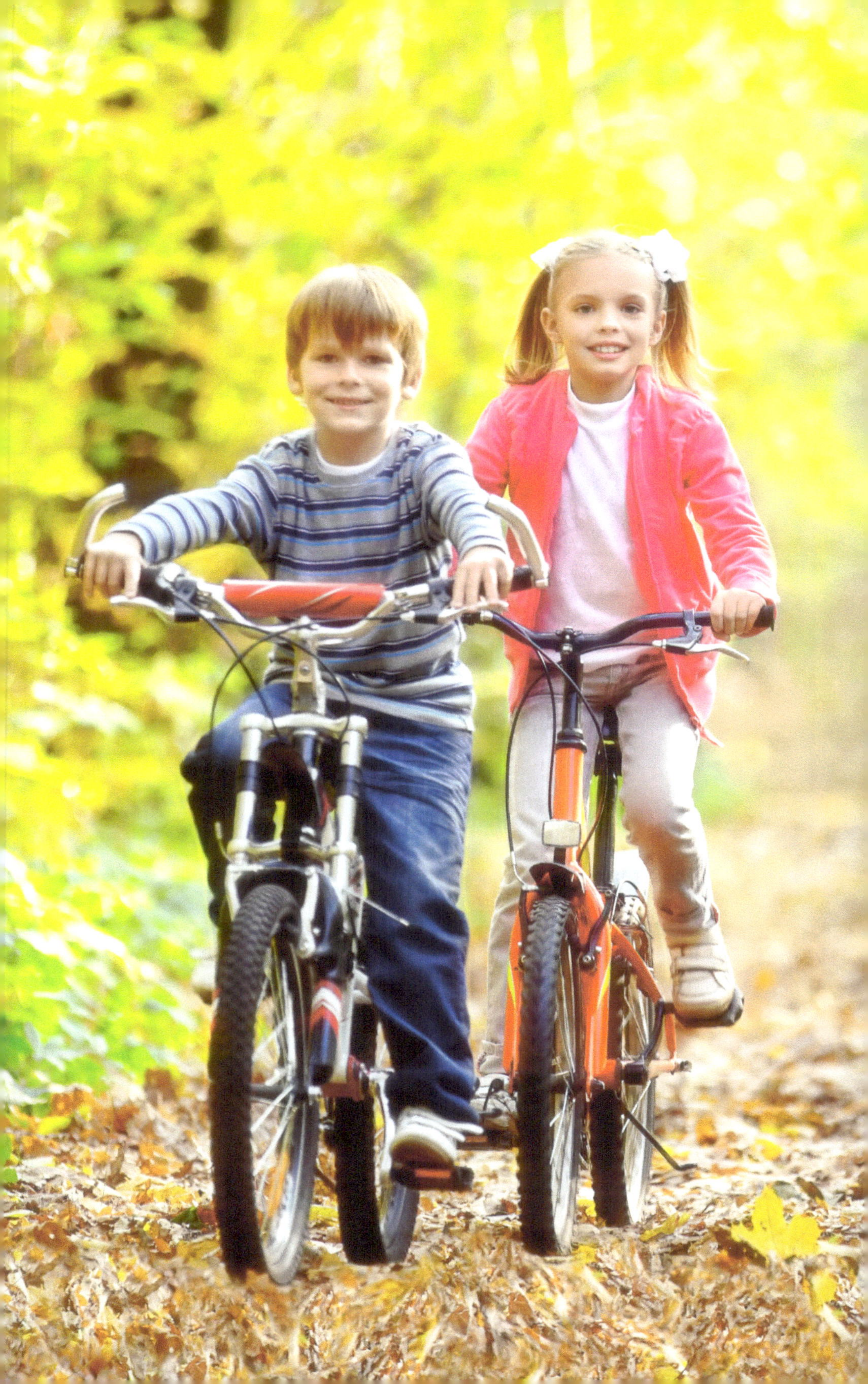

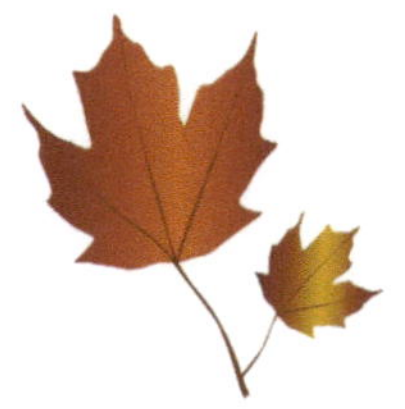

"In the crisp, cool days of autumn, my friends and I loved playing outside. We always went to the forest behind my house because it was the perfect place to play hide and seek."

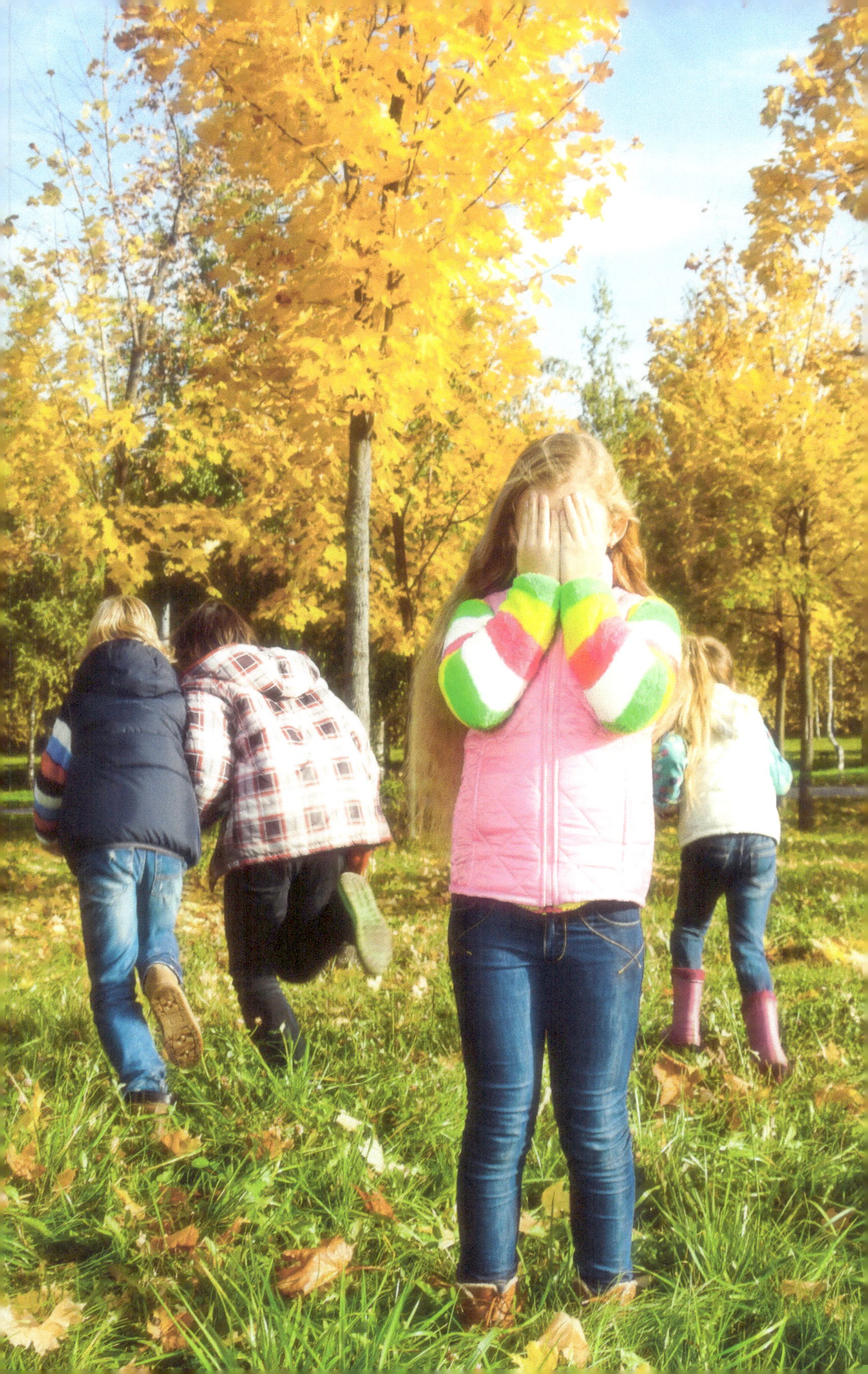

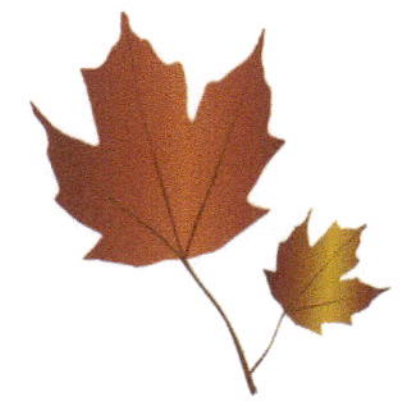

"One cool October day, my parents gave me a pair of rollerblades. Then my Dad took me to the park to teach me how to skate. It wasn't long before I was rolling down the sidewalk all by myself!"

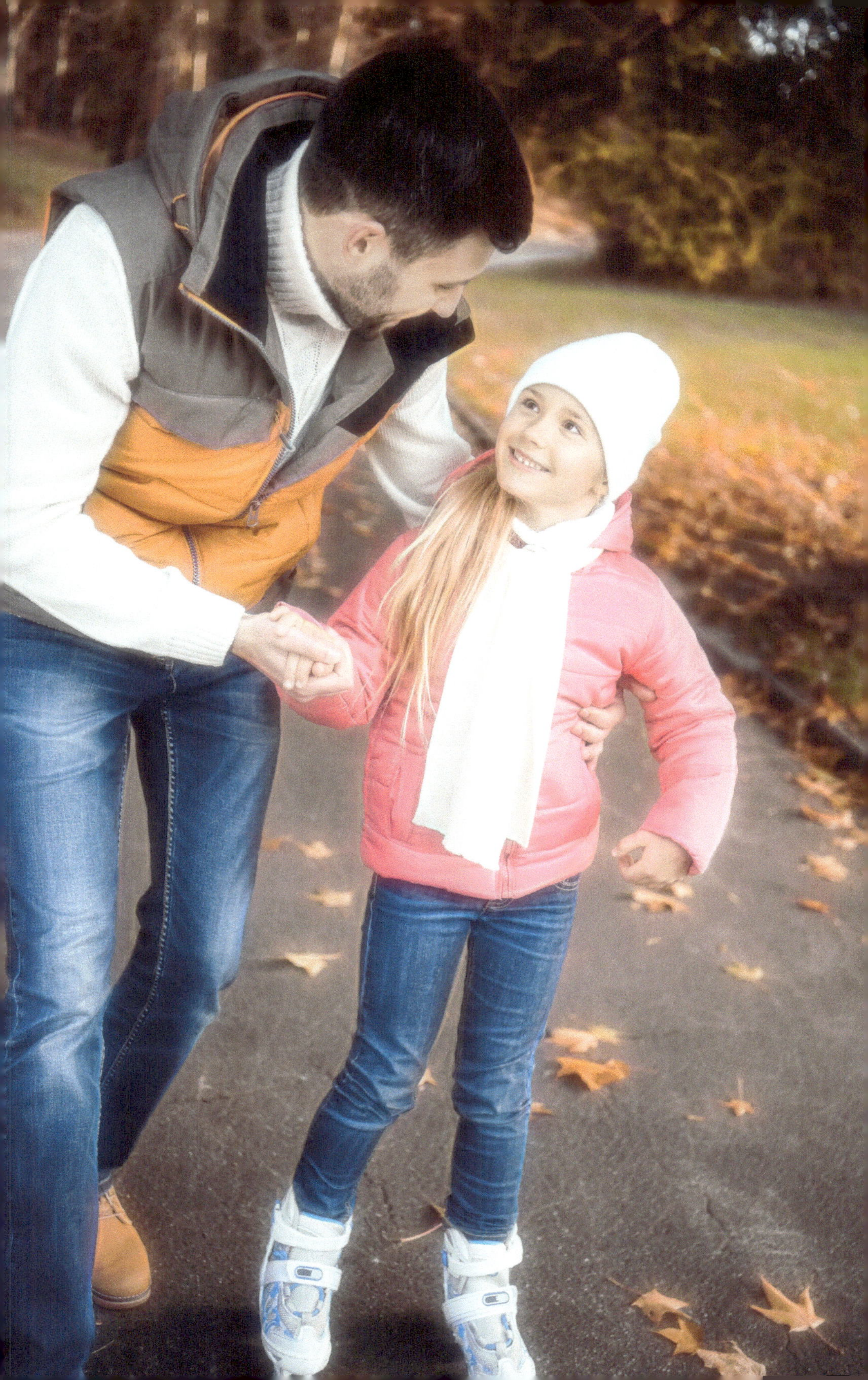

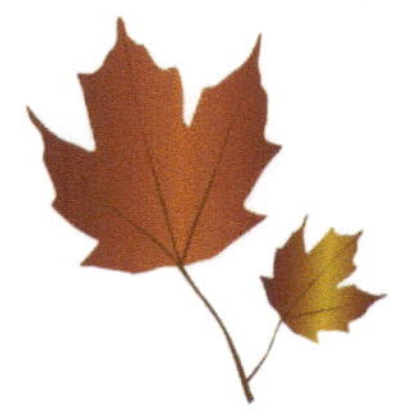

"There was nothing I loved more than going camping with my Dad. My favorite part was starting a campfire so we could toast marshmallows."

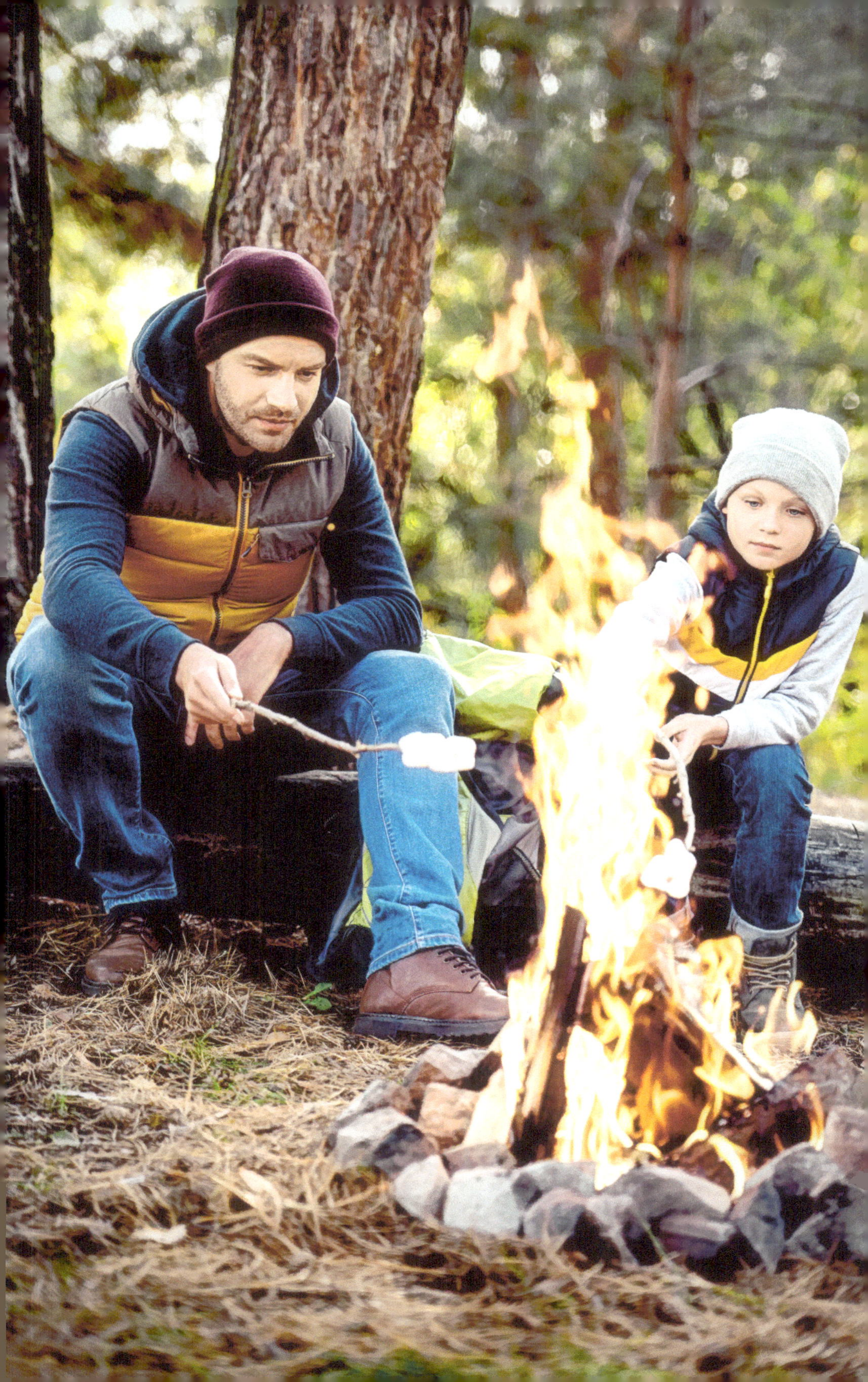

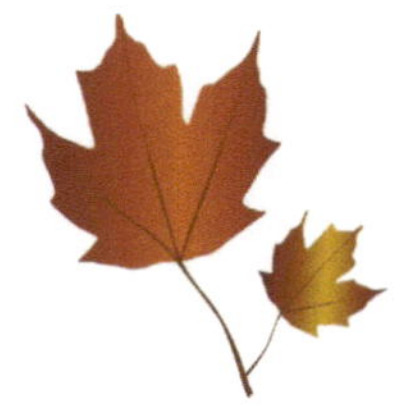

"I loved going to the park to ride my scooter, particularly in autumn. There were so many fallen leaves that the path almost disappeared."

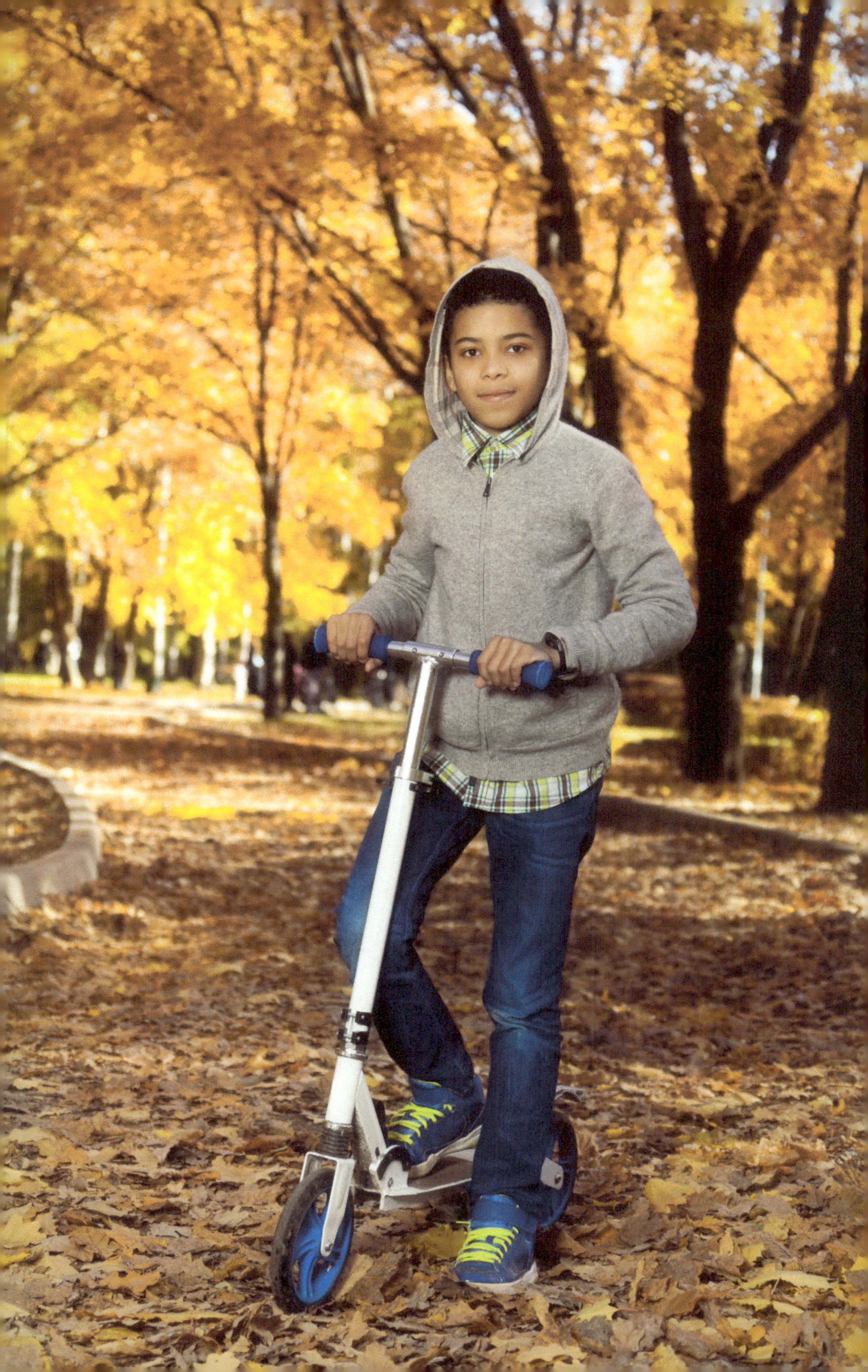

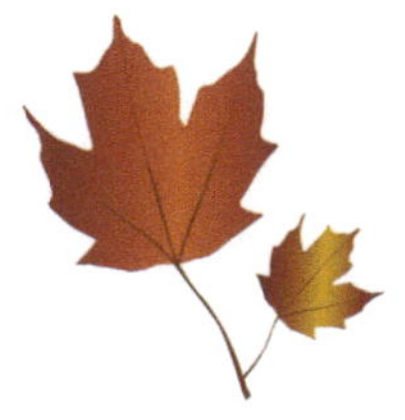

"When the weather turned cool in the autumn, I often went hiking with my parents. They always let me read the map and decide which trail to take."

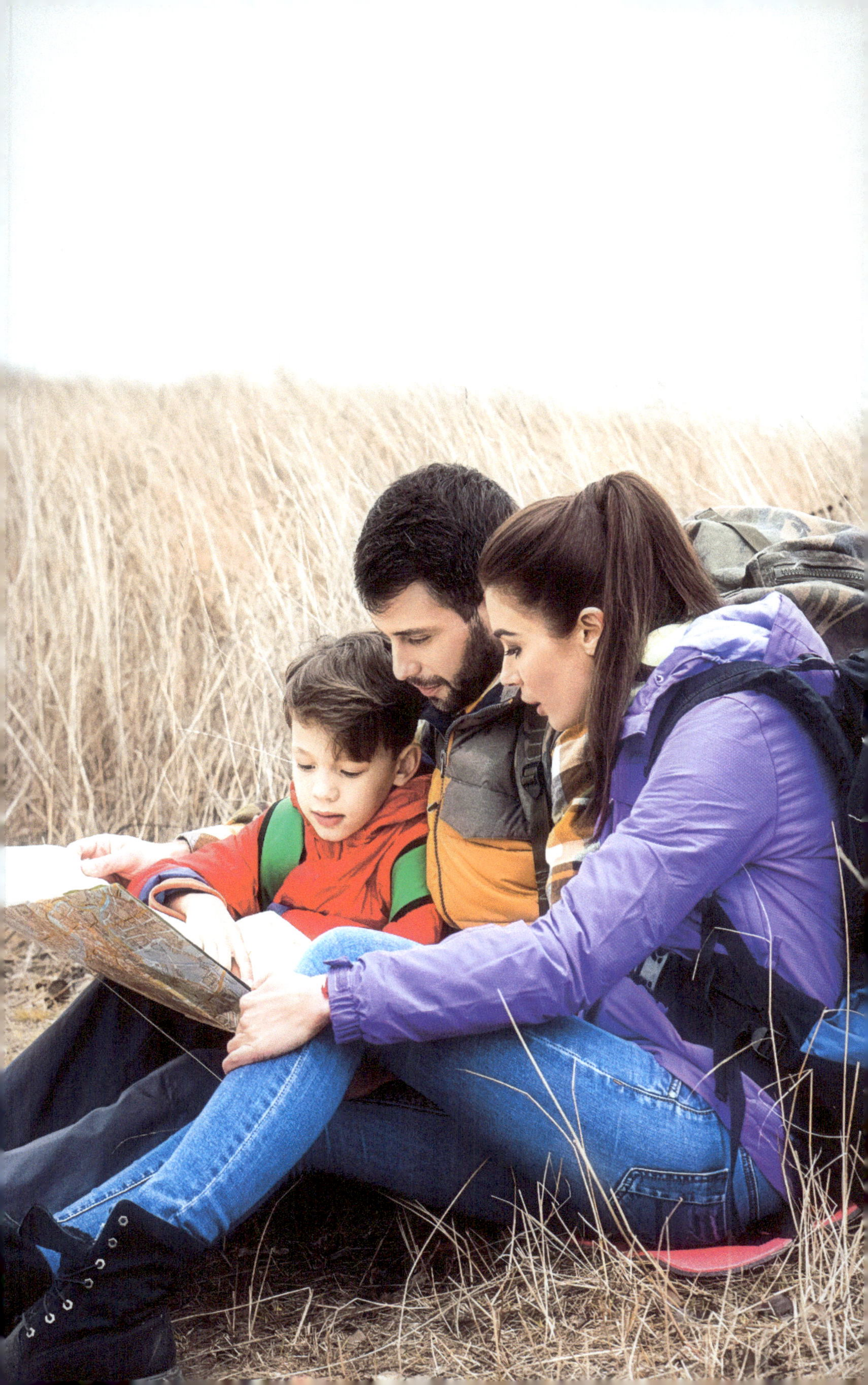

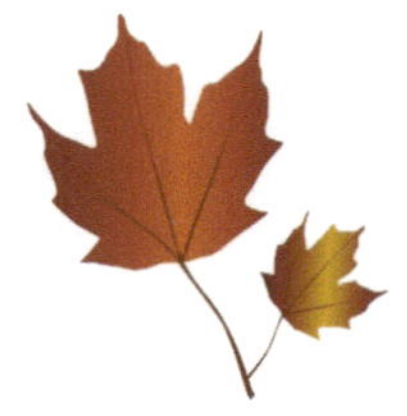

"When I was a kid, I built simple model airplanes and flew them in our backyard, dreaming of the day I'd grow up and become a pilot."

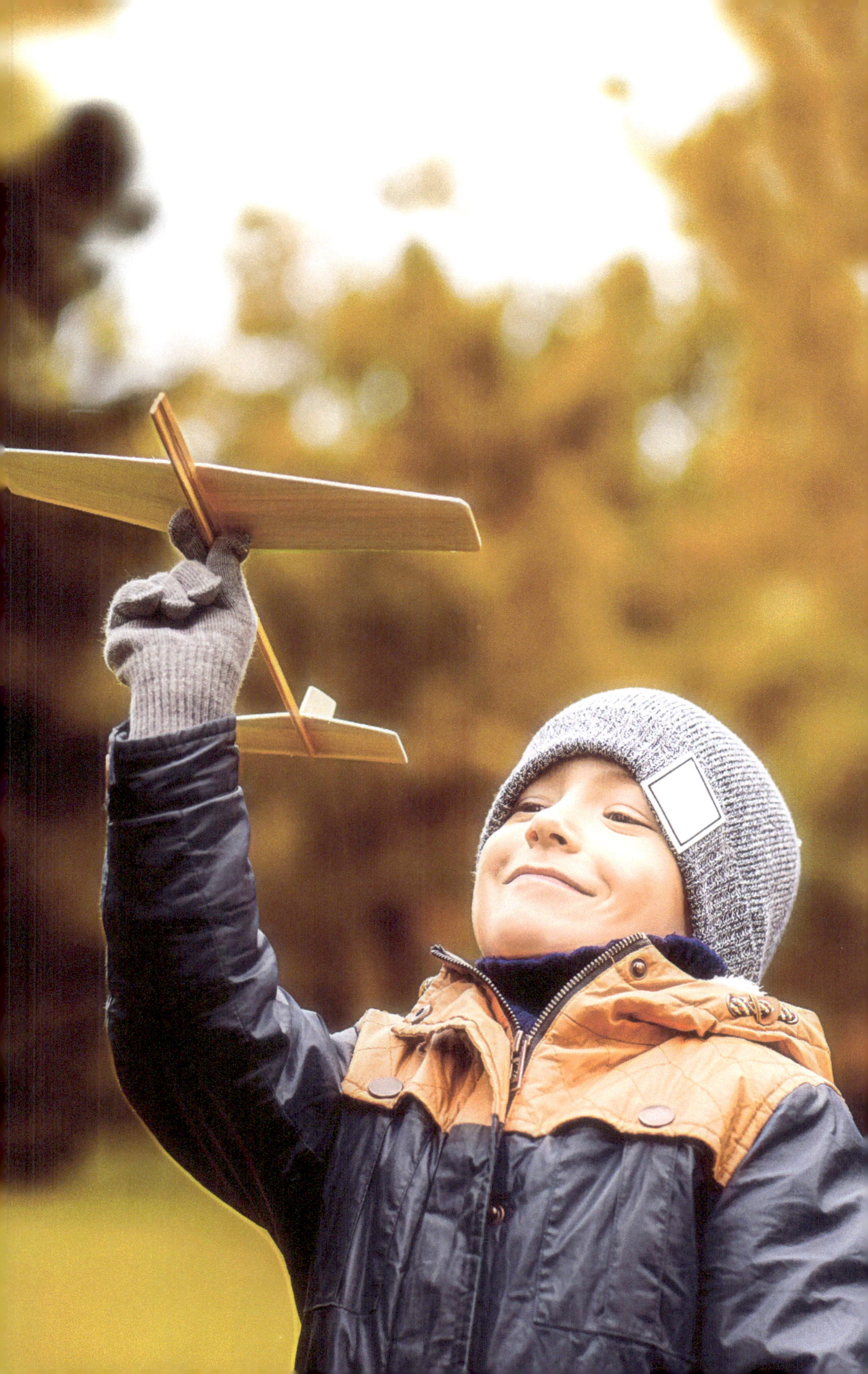

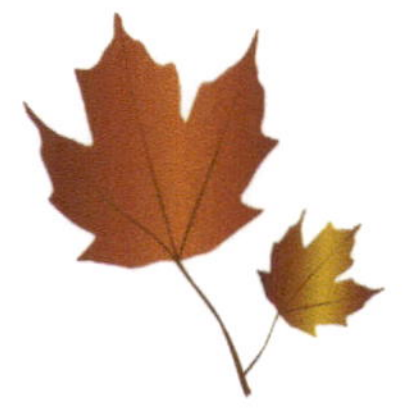

"One weekend when I was eight years old, my family rented a cabin on a beautiful lake. My Mom and I spent a lot of time just sitting on the dock overlooking the lake and talking."

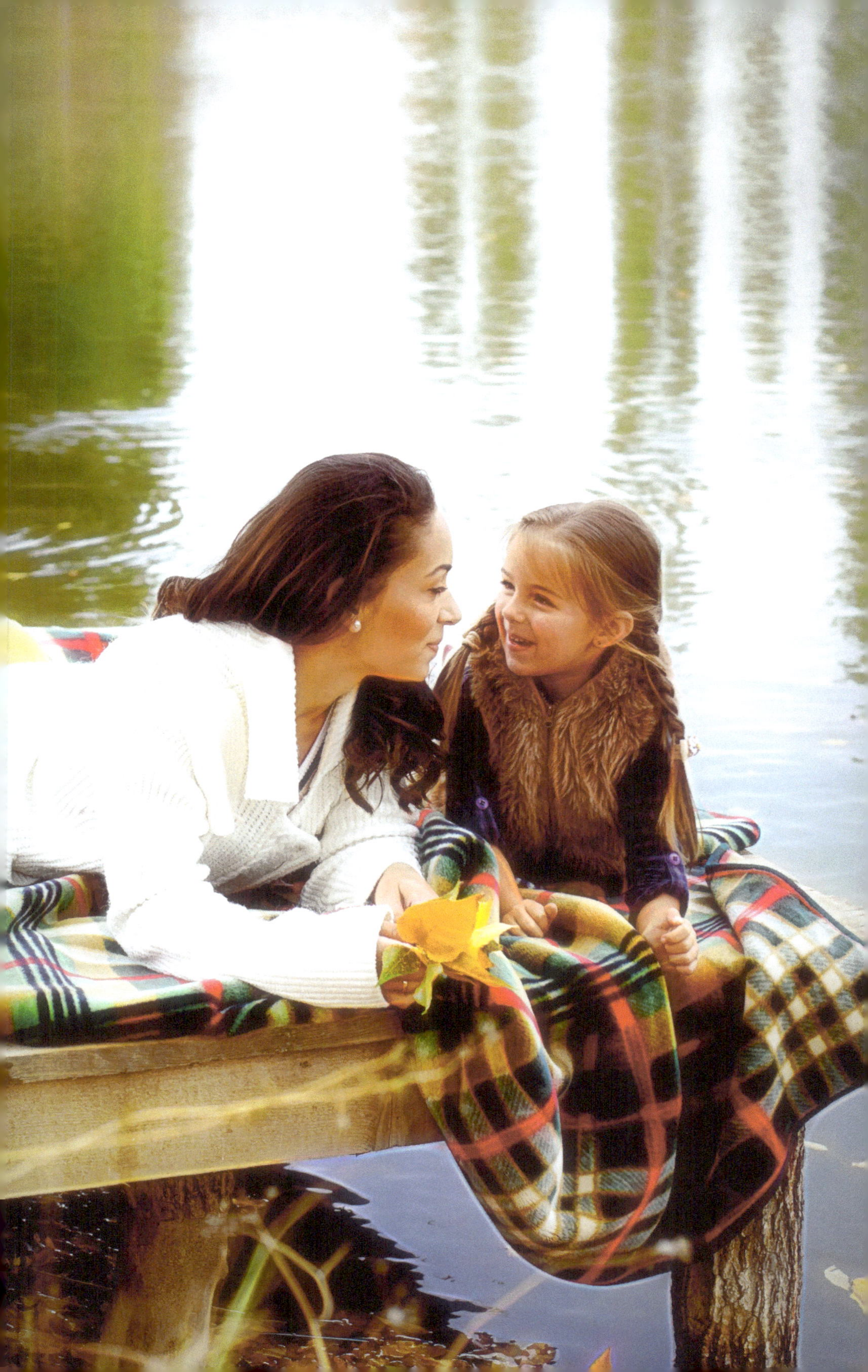

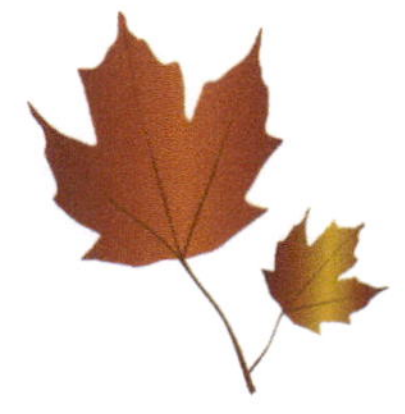

"In late September when I was nine years old, I met a girl who moved into the house next door to ours. She became my best friend. Even now when we're all grown up, we're still best friends."

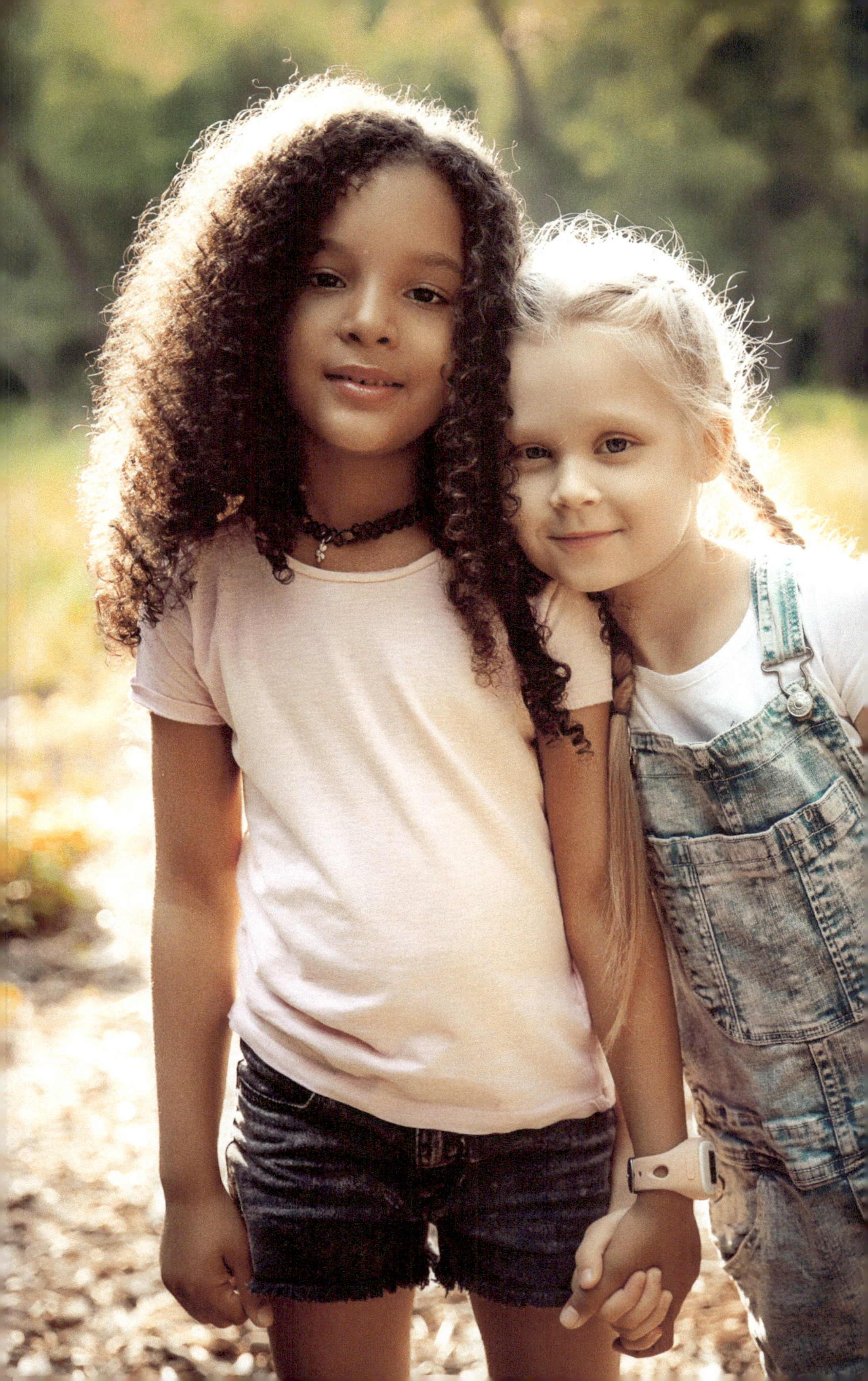

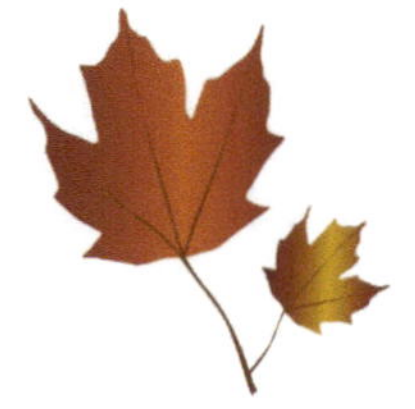

"When autumn came, it was time for the fair! I couldn't wait to ride the rides, play the games, and see the animals. But most of all, I couldn't wait to have some cotton candy!"

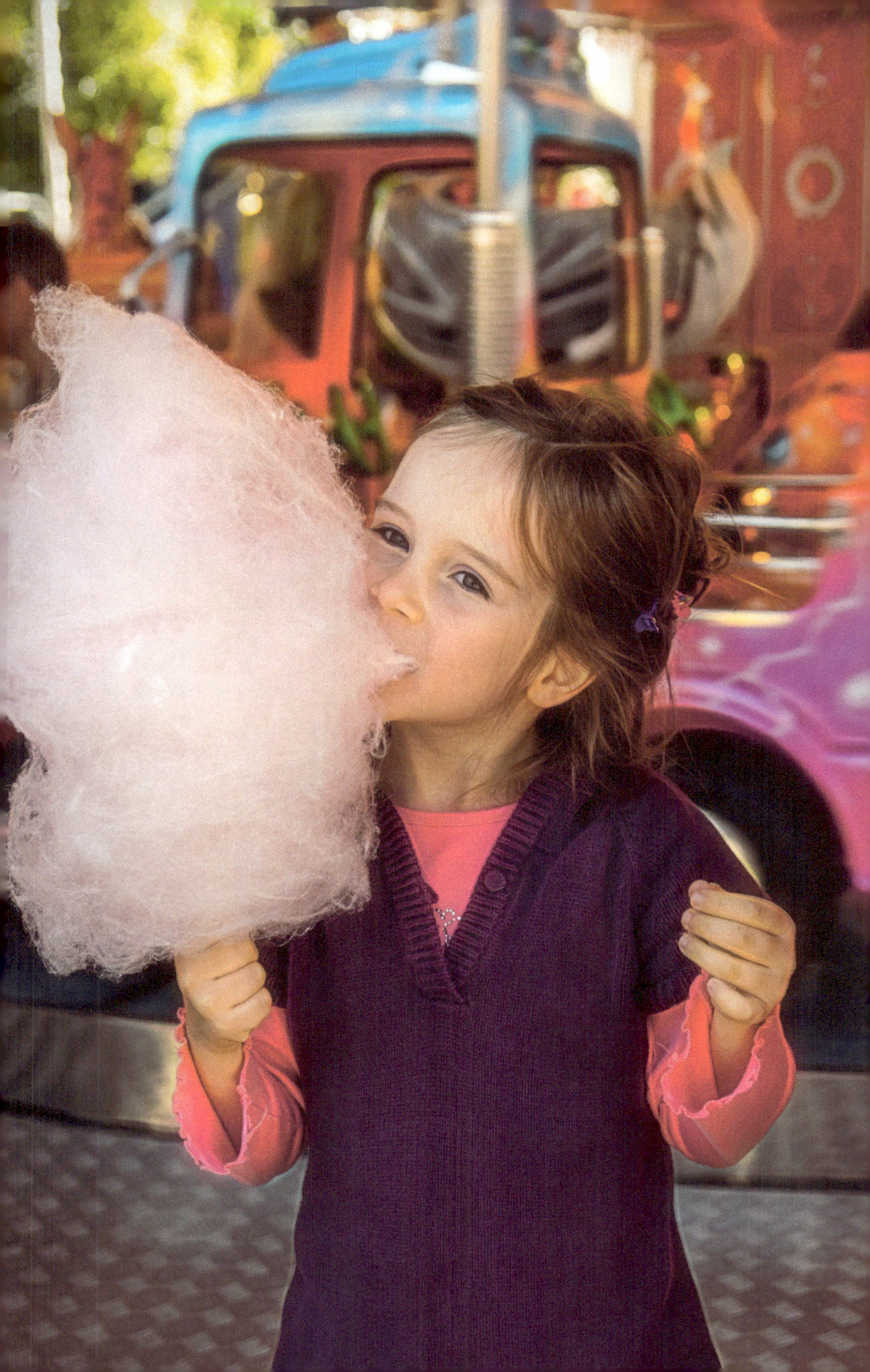

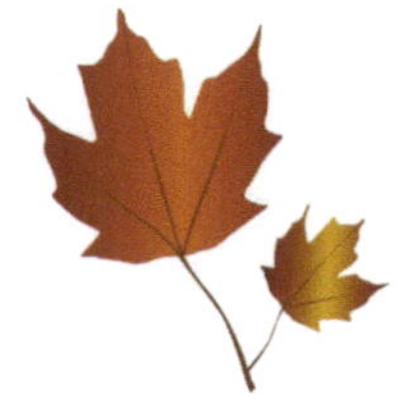

"When I was a kid, there was nothing I loved more than riding my horse. The best time to do it was in the fall, when the air was cool and the trees along the trails were turning beautiful shades of orange and yellow."

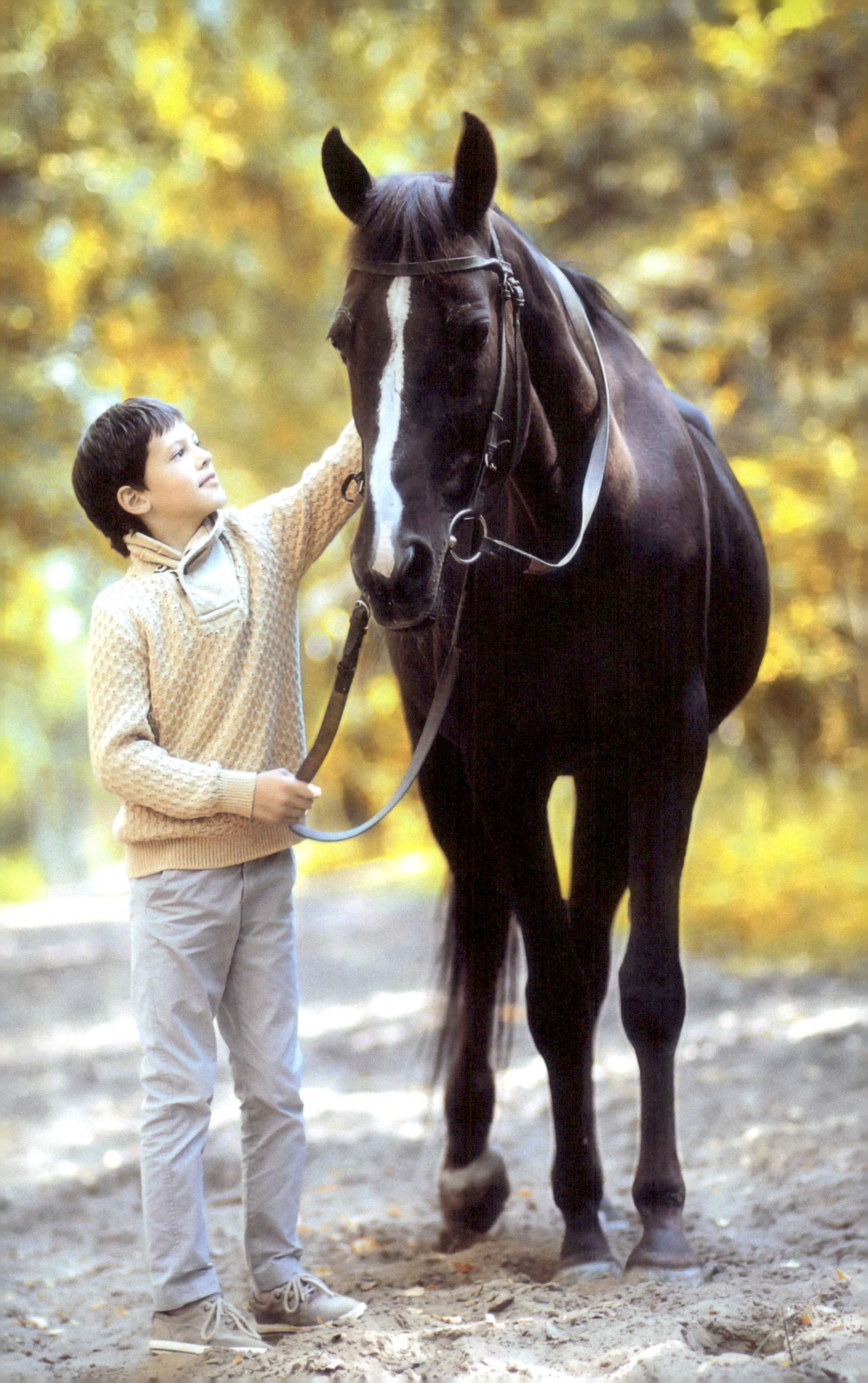

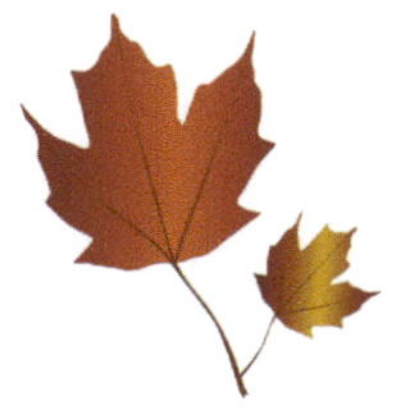

"Around our house, autumn meant one thing--it was time for football! Every Sunday, my Dad and I turned on the television and cheered for our favorite team. I didn't really care if they won or lost. I just liked being with my Dad."

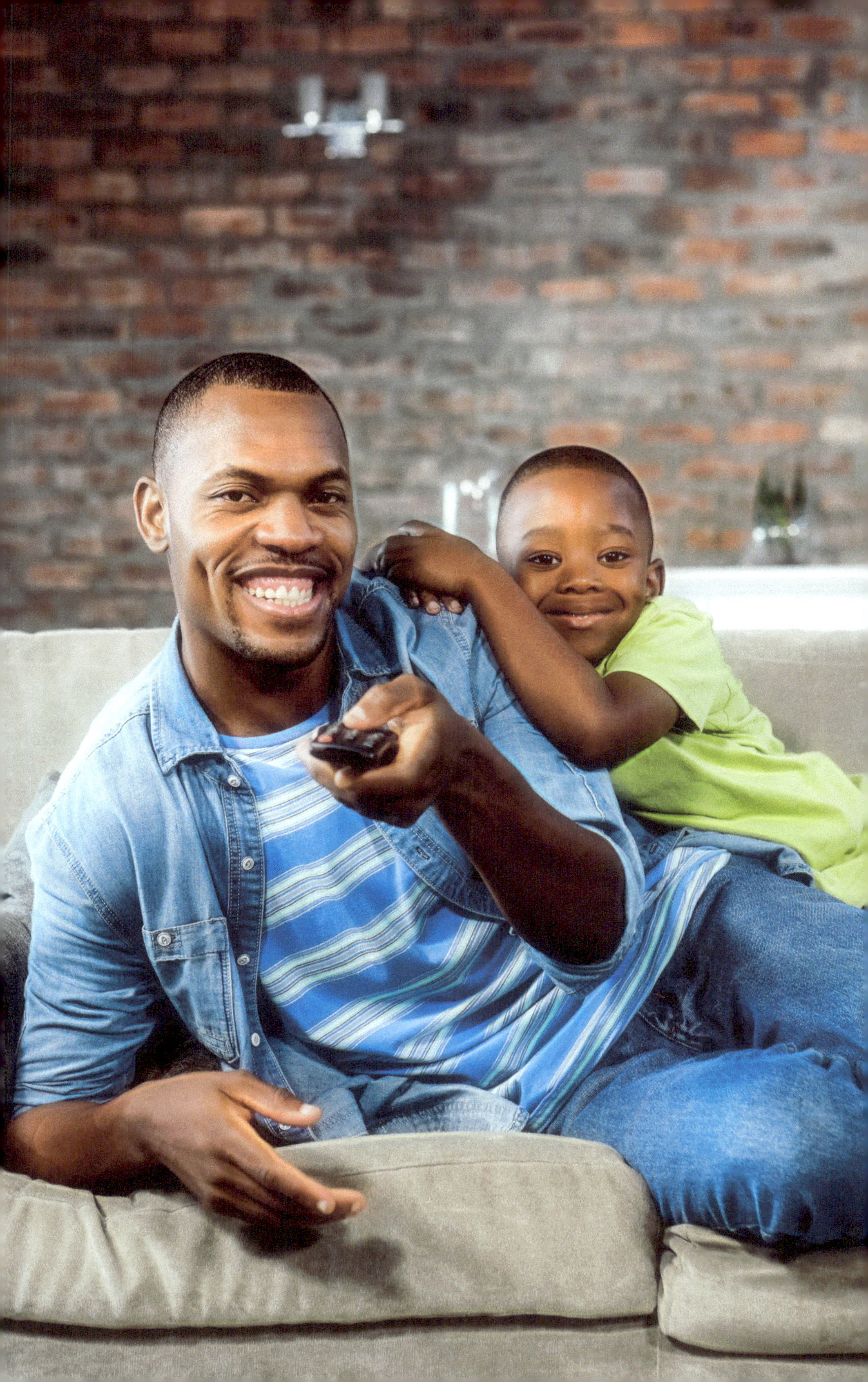

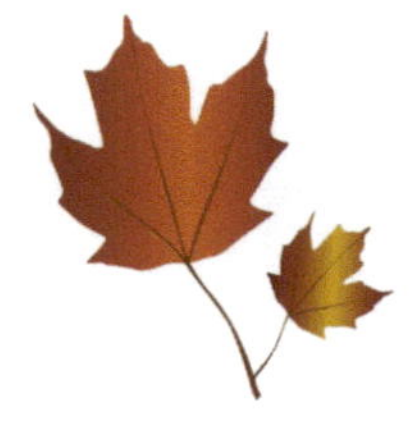

"I always loved it when my Mom read to me. But it felt even more special when the weather turned cold and we could get cozy in front of the fire."

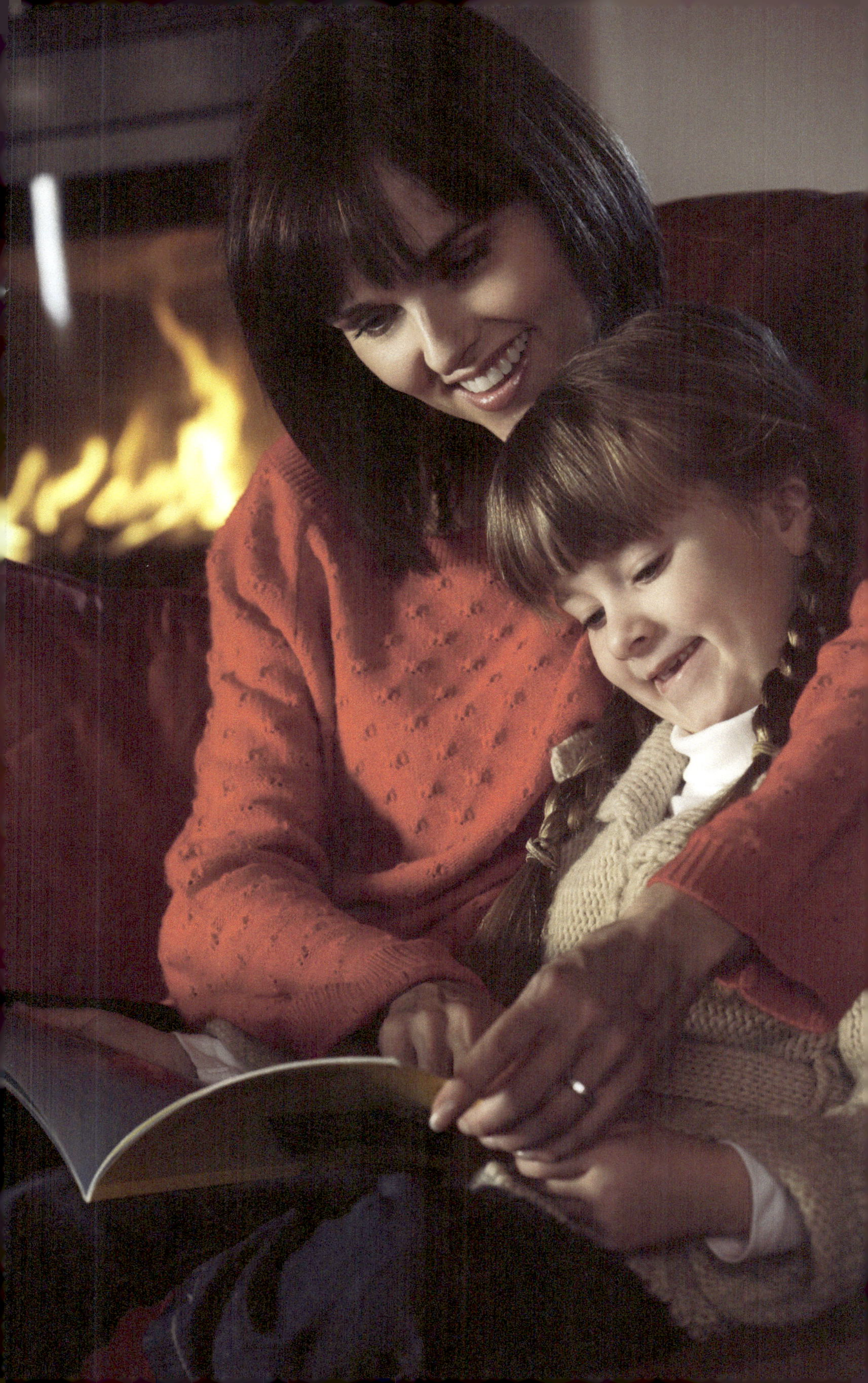